THINGS
I WISH
I'D KNOWN

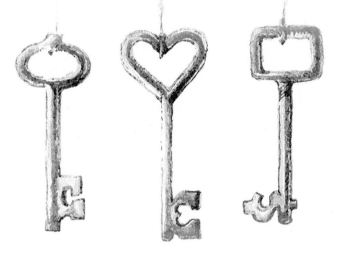

CANCER AND KIDS

Deborah J. Cornwall

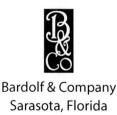

Bardolf & Company
Sarasota, Florida

Bardolf & Company

THINGS I WISH I'D KNOWN
Cancer and Kids

ISBN 978-1-938842-22-1

CIP listing applied for.

Published by Bardolf & Company
5430 Colewood Pl.
Sarasota, FL 34232
941-232-0113
www.bardolfandcompany.com

Cover design and layout by Shaw Creative

Table of Contents

✥ Dedication ✥

*To the more than 35 caregiver interviewees and friends
who shared their stories and experiences
about cancer and children.*

*To those professionals who specialize in supporting
families faced with cancer and in helping them
through the journey and beyond.*

Preface

Most of us shudder when we see the words "cancer" and "kids" in the same sentence. Together they create an unimaginable level of anxiety for parents and other caregivers. It should not be surprising that "How will I tell the kids?" is one of the first questions that a parent or grandparent asks upon hearing a cancer diagnosis.

The coupling of kids and cancer strikes at the core of what parenting means, triggering our instincts to nurture and protect them from harm. Children are supposed to be carefree. They're not supposed to face life-and-death issues among their loved ones, let alone get life-threatening illnesses themselves. When the word "cancer" enters their world, caregivers naturally experience strong reactions, regardless of whether the child is the patient or is part of a household immersed in a cancer battle.

The Cancer Support Community[1], a global network of affiliated nonprofit education and support organizations, estimates that today almost three million children under the age of 18 are living in a household where someone has cancer, and that nearly 600,000 of those have a parent who was diagnosed with cancer within the last two years. This doesn't include the children who themselves or whose siblings received a cancer diagnosis. So if you're a caregiver for a child who fits in one of these categories and are feeling overwhelmed, you're not alone.

This book is drawn from _Things I Wish I'd Known: Cancer Caregivers Speak Out_, which was based on interviews with 95 cancer caregivers for 117 patients who ranged in age from 2 to 92 and experienced the impact of over 40 different cancers on their lives. I have enriched that foundation with dozens of interviews that came about since the second edition of the book was published in 2013, as well as additional research to identify more resources particularly focused on

---

1   www.cancersupportcommunity.org/General-Documents-Category/Newsletters/
     Winter-2013/Program-Spotlight-Kid-Support.htlm

children's issues. Every caregiver who had a child in the family talked of being profoundly touched by the experience of helping the child to understand what was happening to him or someone he loved.

This book offers tips from experts and a variety of resources (with live internet links to tap for more information), as well as compelling stories from people who have experienced the emotional roller coaster involved in helping children to cope with cancer:

Chapter One: Sharing the News

Chapter Two: Managing Cancer's Impact for Children

Chapter Three: When the Child is the Patient

Chapter Four: When Children Lose a Parent or Sibling to Cancer

Chapter Five: Other Resources for Caregivers Concerned About Children

The book will steer you to selected resources for more depth. Resources relevant to particular topics are included in Chapters One through Four, and broader resources are listed in Chapter Five.

One of the most compelling messages from the all of the interviews with family caregivers and social work professionals was that four critical issues dominated their experiences. To help you remember them, I have arranged them so their first letters spell **CHIN**, as in "chin up" or "take it on the chin":

- ∫ **Control:** Loss of control over caregivers' lives was deep-seated and immediate.

- ∫ **Hope:** Their balancing act was the need to maintain hope while at the same time seeking factual information that would help manage both outcomes and expectations.

- ∫ **Isolation:** Most caregivers experienced overwhelming sensations of feeling alone and cut-off, floating in limbo.

- ∫ **Normalcy:** Most mourned for life before cancer. They realized that their lives would never be the same while at the same time aching for things to be as they were before, unaffected by uncertainties or unpredictable turmoil.

As you read, you'll find that the CHIN challenges permeate the book and its caregiver stories.

I know that the caregiving journey with cancer and children is unimaginably difficult. I hope that this little book can provide useful insights and additional support that will ease your mind and help you work through your own situation with more self-confidence and calm.

Deborah J. Cornwall
Marshfield Hills, Massachusetts
January 2015

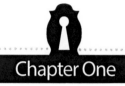

Chapter One

Sharing the News

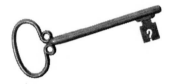

Expert child psychologists and social workers are generally in agreement on key principles for how to discuss cancer with children, regardless of whether a child is the patient or a member of a patient's family. Professionals contend that children are more perceptive than we realize and that the family will be better off with more communication, rather than less.

This chapter will address six important principles you can put into practice:

- **Be Proactive**
- **Tap Experts' Best Guidance**
- **Consult with the Professional Care Team**
- **Meet the Child's Needs, Not Your Own**
- **Level with and Engage Older Children**
- **Be Direct**

While these principles are useful for communicating with all children affected by cancer, additional issues when children themselves are cancer patients are addressed in greater detail in Chapter 3.

Be Proactive

Children sense and will react to changes in a home—your anxious feelings, tired looks, and changes in household routines, whether they're explained or not. And if you don't tell them, they will fill in the void and imagine things that may be far worse than reality.

Tim N's children were 9 and 12 years old when he was diagnosed with cancer at age 42. **Tim N's wife** commented that:

> *Being honest is the only way you can go when you have kids and are faced with cancer, because the kids know what's going on. They didn't even need to overhear something. I'm sure with the phone conversations going on and everyone's dire looks, they knew something was up. To know what it was, they needed some sort of tangible boundaries put on the thing so they could understand it and put it in its place.*

In another home where a parent had been diagnosed with cancer, an 11-year-old saw the caller-ID on the phone when the cancer center called.

The reality is that you'll need to tell the kids something, so getting the topic out in the open is enormously helpful. Fred Rogers,[2] whose television show, *Mr. Rogers' Neighborhood*, ran for many years on Public Broadcasting System, had an ease in communicating with children. He believed that opening the door when you hear an unexpected noise on the other side and seeing what's behind it is healthier than keeping the door closed:

> *Anything that's human is mentionable, and anything that is mentionable can be more manageable. When we can talk about our feelings, they become less overwhelming, less upsetting, and less scary. The people we trust with that important talk can help us know that we are not alone.[3]*

A child whose concerns are trapped inside, who hasn't had the opportunity to learn what's going on and may be building up fear and anxiety, can become

---

2 http://pbskids.org/rogers/
3 http://www.goodreads.com/author/quotes/32106.Fred_Rogers

emotionally fragile and express pent-up feelings in a variety of ways. Depending on age, that could be bed-wetting or thumb-sucking, complaints of stomach upset, nightmares, anger or irritability, withdrawal from habitual activities, or even risk-taking behaviors like bullying or drinking.

When you open up channels of communication with children about cancer facing the family, they might become emotional, angry, or a little moody, but they won't break. It's better to have a safe pressure valve for relieving uncomfortable feelings with someone they can trust, rather than waiting for them to act out with destructive or risky behavior.

Tap Experts' Best Guidance

Determining what to say to children when a parent, sibling, or close relative has cancer is always a sensitive decision because you're trying to explain that things are different while at the same time trying not to scare them. Depending on age and maturity, each needs a different type and amount of information. Each will digest information at a different rate, but all need open communication.

One of the best resources to help with that is by Martha Aschenbrenner, a child life specialist with MD Anderson's Supportive Care Program. Her _Comprehensive Guide: Child Life From Another Perspective_,[4] is available online in PDF form. The 20-page document offers simple insights about how to discuss a diagnosis and its implications with children.

One of its most important contributions is the concept of the three Cs:

- ๑ The illness is called Cancer.

- ๑ It is not Catchy (or Contagious).

- ๑ It is not Caused by anything the child did or did not do.

These three principles demonstrate honesty and anticipate the kinds of concerns that the child might have (Will I get it, too? Will you? Was it my fault?). The guide also provides a variety of useful metaphors and visual images

---

4 _www.mdanderson.org/patient-and-cancer-information/guide-to-md-anderson/patient-and-family-support/child-life-journal.pdf_

that can be helpful in talking with children of varying ages about what cancer is and what to expect.

Another excellent guide is the pamphlet _Frankly Speaking About Cancer: What Do I Tell the Kids?_[5] published by The Cancer Support Community. This invaluable booklet (also available online) is an important starting point that addresses issues and comprehension by age level.

Still another useful resource is the _Parenting at a Challenging Time_ (PACT)[6] program that was developed at the Massachusetts General Hospital and is now offered in several other hospitals nationwide. The website for the program provides helpful information about how to talk with children.

More comprehensive information can be accessed in _Raising an Emotionally Healthy Child When a Parent is Sick_ (A Harvard Medical School Book),[7] written by Paula K. Rauch, M.D., founder and director of the PACT program, and Anna C. Muriel, M.D., M.P.H., member of the PACT staff.

For families dealing with childhood cancers, the _Children's Cancer Research Fund_ has a list of books[8] for helping kids to understand cancer and serious illnesses. In addition, the site offers insights about pediatric cancer research as well as stories of children who have survived serious cancer bouts.

Finally, the _American Childhood Cancer Organization_[9] provides a variety of free books for children with cancer and their families, as well as what they call a Treatment Kit (also free) that includes a duffle bag, fleece blanket, pillow case, and pack of playing cards. The books include journals for parents, adolescents, and children for recording their feelings and thoughts as treatment proceeds. Two of those books for children are available in Spanish.

All of these resources give you options, but all are targeted at helping to meet the children, age-appropriately, wherever they are in their need and readiness for information.

---

5   _www.amazon.com/Raising-Emotionally-Healthy-Harvard-Medical/dp/0071446818_
6   _www.mghpact.org/for-parents/parents_
7   _www.amazon.com/Raising-Emotionally-Healthy-Harvard-Medical/dp/0071446818_
8   _www.childrenscancer.org/main/books_for_helping_kids_deal_with_cancer/_
9   _www.acco.org/Information/Resources/Books.aspx_

Consult with the Professional Care Team

Comprehensive cancer centers for adults and children are growing more sensitive to these issues: if they haven't yet built sophisticated consulting teams to help adult patients tell children about cancer, plans for doing so are probably on the drawing board. Resources cited earlier in this chapter are invaluable, but nothing compares with a personal conversation with trained professionals who know the patient and family situation. You'll be wise to seek them out to help you engage children in the conversation in an age-appropriate way that will enrich them and every member of the family.

Meet the Child's Needs, Not Your Own

Experts say you should plan proactive communication with children who will be affected by cancer, because unlike most adults, they have fewer resources (fewer contacts, information, or life experience) to make sense of ambiguity and uncertainty. What's hard, though, is imagining a conversation with children about cancer before you're sure what you're thinking and feeling yourself. That's why getting your own head in gear (as discussed in Chapter Two) is a prerequisite to talking with the children. Otherwise you risk getting them more alarmed than might be necessary or appropriate.

The urge to protect children, and indirectly to protect yourself from uncomfortable and unpredictable questions, is hard to overcome. For some people, this can be unsettling. After all, aren't parents supposed to have the answers? Won't the kids feel upset if I can't tell them what will be happening over time?

The professionals and caregivers who shared such stories all recommended:

- ◡ Telling the truth (adjusted to the children's age and maturity).
- ◡ Managing their expectations so they can prepare themselves for what's to come.
- ◡ Encouraging them to sustain their routine activities and to maintain as much normalcy in their interactions with the patient as possible.

In your zeal to communicate, though, remember to be sensitive to the child's ability to understand and digest what you're saying.

Rob, age 29, was in the midst of a chondroid chordoma diagnosis during the ramp-up to Christmas. His young children had observed the flurry of unusual activity and suspected that it wasn't holiday-related. **Rob's wife** described how they handled it:

> They could sense that something was different because I was on the computer all the time. The night before the biopsy I said, "Daddy has something in his head that doesn't belong there. The doctors are going to take a look and figure out what it is. When he gets home, he'll be tired, but he will still be your same dad." One of them asked, "Is Daddy going to die?" We had agreed ahead of time that we had to be honest, so I told them that as soon as we knew more, we'd tell them more.

The conversation needs to be kid-centric and to allow for many follow-up talks. Prepare them for the most obvious changes they'll see in the patient who may become easily upset, be too tired to play, go to frequent medical appointments, lose his or her hair, and so on. The conversations are an opportunity to model for children how to communicate about sensitive subjects. Your open sharing at appropriate levels of information will build trust that you will tell them if something changes and that they can raise any questions or concerns with you.

Always remember: the conversation isn't about you and what you need to express; it's about the children and what they need to hear.

Be Direct

Medical treatments are unpredictable in terms of how a particular patient's cancer will respond or progress. So when you do discuss a family member's cancer, you won't be able to be definitive about longer term outcomes. On the other hand, most younger children won't need that right away. Usually they're about the "now." They will need to know about:

☙ **What will be different in the household and why.** Identify the illness. When you name cancer, you're conveying that you'll be honest and direct, rather than beating around the bush with euphemisms like "Daddy is sick."

☙ **How you plan to keep things as close to normal as you can.** Your children's concerns will be fairly immediate and practical, and nowhere near as long-term or "cosmic" as your own. They will want to know what it means for changes in day-to-day routines. Who will be home when I get off the bus? Will Grandma still be able to be with us for the holidays? Can I keep going to swimming practice?

☙ **What other people may be called on for help** (Yes, you'll need a team for support). Be clear about whom you'll call on to maintain schedules and routines in the household.

☙ **Treatment plans.** Since experienced doctors and nurses have a treatment plan for the person with cancer, children need to know it exists and the basic terms.

☙ **Your commitment to ongoing conversation.** Ask children to tell you what they might be wondering about, and don't be surprised if they don't have any questions or want to talk right away. Children process information by cycling in and out of new topics. One minute they'll be immersed in the conversation and the next they'll be off, interacting with friends or engaged in their regular activities. That's their sign to you that they've had enough for now, not a sign of disinterest.

Dealing with the unknown can be the most difficult thing for younger children, so it helped Ellen W's eight-year-old daughter to meet the hospital social worker and to see where her mom was receiving chemotherapy. **Ellen W's husband** explained that:

> We keep it as light as we can. "Mom's going to the hospital." Our daughter knows it's cancer but we tell her that the doctors are doing all the right stuff to make mommy better. No odds or anything. We brought her in to watch Ellen get chemo, and our social worker

15

took her around and gave her a tour of the medical oncologist's office area, so he and she are buddies now. Frankly, our daughter finds it all a little boring.

Ellen and her husband engaged their daughter verbally and in other ways that let her see where her mother was going so often. Just the fact that she found it boring demonstrates that they managed to minimize for her the turmoil and sense of drama that they were experiencing.

Remember: Not every question needs an immediate and detailed response. If you don't know how to respond, tell the children that you might want to consult someone and will let them know what you find out.

Level With and Engage Older Children

Older children often pose even more of a challenge than younger ones. Little ones often guide you with the questions they ask; they let you know how much they are ready to hear. Older children may profess to want total truth but aren't always ready to hear it, so their parents can help them by minimizing the resulting disruption in their lives. There are no easy answers about how to reach a good balance.

In general, as with younger children, caregivers suggest telling older children the truth but in this case adjusting the message to the severity of the diagnosis. The most difficult challenge is managing their expectations in situations where the outcome is unknown because older children have more life experience and are quick to project alternative results.

When James was diagnosed with incurable multiple myeloma, he and his wife decided to inform their children, who were in the same college, during a pre-scheduled parents' weekend five weeks later. **James' wife** explained:

We wanted to tell them in person. It's hard to tell your kids that their father has incurable cancer. We had discussed it and didn't want the kids feeling they needed to come home every weekend. So we decided to tell them the good, the bad, and the ugly so they wouldn't worry that things were being hidden or held back.

We kept to that game plan. They asked what the doctor had said, and we said he'd have two to three years with standard treat-

ments, but we've learned about new stuff, especially bone mar-
row transplants, that could make it better. Information was a
tool for them as well. The kids were comforted by knowing that
we'd told them everything.

That was over 23 years ago. As of this writing, James continues to thrive.

When caregivers limit information sharing to the point where a parent's death comes as a shock to the older children, it is not unusual for them to remain angry afterwards—in some cases for years—because they were not included.

That's what happened when **Lynn's husband** followed the wishes of his wife to manage the flow of information to their college-age children and keep the news cheerful. When she died, they were in shock because they had had so little warning:

Our son was in Manhattan, and our daughter in Belgium. She
was finishing her master's degree there, and it had been Lynn's
preference for her not to keep running home. We gave them
thumbnails which were always positive and hopeful. In fact,
things were upbeat until three days before she died. After the
funeral, our daughter was upset and said, "You didn't tell me
the truth!"

There is no easy answer about how to handle such a situation. Sometimes the healthy parent will need to think it through and decide that doing something other than what the patient requested is the best solution for the child's future emotional well-being.

Above all, be kind to yourself. Life is about making choices, and in an unpredictable and serious cancer situation, there are no easy decisions in managing the information flow to children of any age. Ultimately, all you can do is make the best possible decision under the circumstances. Show love to all concerned but with eyes open to the potential negative consequences, and be prepared to work through those consequences after the fact.

Chapter Two

Managing Cancer's Impact for Children

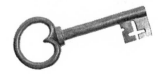

Managing the impact of cancer on children's lives centers on three key principles:

- ৶ **Seek Out Professional Resources**
- ৶ **Maintain Normalcy in Household Routines: Build a Team to Help**
- ৶ **Let Children Participate in Care**

Seek Out Professional Resources

As you think about gathering support for yourself in your role as caregiver, you may want to consider enrolling your children in programs geared specifically for helping them deal with the impact of cancer in their family. Such programs can help them overcome their sense of isolation, the feeling that they are the only ones in the world who feel as they do.

The Cancer Support Community[10] offers an evidence-based program called Kid Support™ in many of its 46 U.S. affiliates. It provides a place for kids

---

10   *www.cancersupportcommunity.org*

between the ages of 4 and 16 to interact, learn about cancer and its treatments, validate their emotions, reduce their feelings of isolation and loss of control, and cope with loss of normalcy. Participating children have been able to reduce cancer-related stress by learning communication and relaxation skills, gaining age-appropriate knowledge, and engaging in dialogue and activities with other cancer-impacted children. The program (which is offered in many CSC locations, free of charge) brings kids together weekly and conducts parent meetings every other week, with the goal of increasing family dialogue and reducing family stress.

Another type of helpful resource to help children process what they hear about cancer in the family uses expressive arts (image making, writing, sound, and movement). Laura Tryon Jennings, a trained expressive arts facilitator, who works specifically with art, says that group activities focusing on discussion alone may be important to provide some children with a break from focusing on cancer. Others may benefit from learning how to convert their negative emotions into more peaceful feelings and constructive behaviors by using more than just words to express themselves:

> In one group, I was working with two children who had lost a sibling to cancer several months before. Their mother had brought them because they were showing anger and frustration that was disruptive both in school and at home. I invited them to use black and red chalk to draw on paper whatever they were feeling. After a few hesitant moments, they dove into the exercise, fiercely scribbling away and making a variety of sounds, coloring the paper and even their bodies. Afterward they said they felt terrific. Their mother said she hadn't seen them smile in seven months and that this exercise had triggered a behavioral breakthrough.

Similar programs may be available from a nearby cancer center or from a community organization in your city. Ask your cancer center's patient navigator or oncology social worker to help you find such a program near you.

Maintain Normalcy in Household Routines: Build a Team to Help

Try to keep the mechanics of day-to-day living as predictable as possible. This may require getting others involved to help. Ensure that the children know every day what will be happening and who will be managing their activities. Assemble a team around you (including representatives from school) so that the caregiving roller coaster that you're on won't turn their daily routines or behavior topsy-turvy.

When Mindy was undergoing chemotherapy for a potentially fatal metastatic melanoma without a primary site, her oncologist reminded the couple that they might feel they were losing control of their lives but that they could still control how they cared for their children. Carrying out that guidance, **Mindy's husband** maintained normalcy for three children of disparate ages by mobilizing a team to help manage the daily logistics:

> *You have to create a community of helpers if you don't have one. Pick out the most difficult time of day. For me, it's morning, because getting three kids of different ages ready for school takes two adults. At 6 a.m. every day my mother is here, every school day. She lives 7 minutes away, and we live close enough to the elementary school to walk or ride a bike. We kept the baby with someone she knew.*
>
> *Our parents were a massive help. It's incredibly hard to care for a toddler, elementary school kid, and a middle schooler, each with different needs, from 4:30 to 9 pm. That was the hardest time for me. The two moms switched off in the evenings.*
>
> *I asked the school counselor to treat our 13-year-old as if she was his mother when he was at school. We told her that we couldn't influence what happens at school, so she should do whatever she felt was professionally and motherly the right thing to do. We told her she had absolute latitude to do it.*

A critical part of maintaining normalcy is devising ways for children to continue their usual activities interacting with other children. This means that you or other team members may need to orchestrate play dates, sleepovers, movie dates, sports games, and so on. It's important to give children respites from being surrounded by cancer 24/7 and for them to have fun.

Let Children Participate in Care

Children can bring joy in many ways, especially by just being themselves. Most of us have experienced how a child's giggle can make us laugh, or how a hug or an adoring look can warm our hearts. Another great thing about kids is that they lack the self-consciousness that sometimes causes adults to pull away from a cancer patient. For them, you are who you are, even if you don't have hair, are on oxygen, or are feeling queasy. The impact of their presence can be profoundly positive for a cancer patient.

When Susan was diagnosed with a terminal brain tumor, her daughter Stacey was pregnant, and Susan was given the opportunity to interact with the baby right after he was born. **Stacey's sister Kim** explained that:

> *Stacey had labor induced so Mom could be there at the birth. They put her in a chair that was convertible to a bed. When she'd get tired, she'd lie down next to Stacey. We put her in a wheelchair when Stacey gave birth. She was the first to hold the baby. He was a little bundle of joy for her. We'd wrap him up and she would hold him in bed. We'd joke that it was her turn to watch him. So she was a part of it. It brought a sense of normalcy. He was her first grandson after having had four granddaughters.*

Mike S's wife said that her husband found that the active involvement and unselfishness of their older children in his care enriched and greatly improved the quality of his life:

> *Our son Josh would cook things he thought might appeal to Mike. He was never discouraged when Mike ate only a spoonful. Josh also participated in the direct caregiving, initially just as a companion. Later, Josh picked up nursing skills, helping Mike with dressing, hydration, and so on. I think the physical touching involved in helping his father do daily things was important. Men and male children are less likely to touch each other or to hug.*

Our other son, Jonah, would settle in with Mike to watch sports in the evening, though neither of them was a particularly avid sport fan. Mike could be on the couch and doze off. When he woke up, Jonah would give him the score and an update. It gave them time together doing something they wouldn't ordinarily have done.

For some families the daily routine can be a welcome distraction from cancer. **Jen P's husband** explained that despite her treatment schedule:

We had little kids who needed what little kids need, and we didn't have time to sit around and mope and feel sorry for ourselves because day-to-day life things didn't stop for us. Diapers and naps. They needed us. It was helpful—it forced us to take our minds off ourselves because there were others depending on us for their lives.

It is important to find ways to maintain children's ordinary family lives while also letting them interact in normal fashion with the person who has cancer, be it a sibling, parent, grandparent, or close family friend. Similarly, as discussed in the next chapter, it is critical for children who are cancer patients themselves to be able to sustain their relationships with their family members and friends to help carry them through difficult treatments.

Part of participating in care is letting them be themselves in their dealings with the cancer patient. Every patient seeks normalcy, and children can help remind them of life before cancer struck.

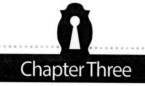

Chapter Three

When the Child is the Patient

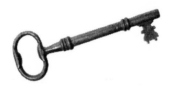

It shouldn't come as a surprise that a cancer diagnosis for a child puts parents through an emotional wringer. As Michel L's mother said of her learning about her nine-year-old son's brain tumor:

> *"Cancer" is a taboo word. It never comes into your mind when your child is sick. When they told me, I couldn't see or hear anything. My mind was racing.*

Almost all of the parental caregivers described how a child's serious cancer diagnosis provoked such intense feelings of profound helplessness, it was hard to maintain the focus, stability, and calm required to make rational caregiving decisions and to advocate effectively with medical providers.

This chapter addresses nine topics to keep in mind as you're dealing with a childhood cancer diagnosis:

- **Get Your Head in Gear**
- **Pin Down and Understand the Diagnosis Fast**
- **Seek the Best Treatments**
- **Conserve Your Energy**
- **Advocate during Treatment**

- ∽ **Head Off Needle Phobia in Very Young Children**
- ∽ **Fight Isolation**
- ∽ **Plan for Survivorship Issues**
- ∽ **When the Child's Diagnosis is Grim:**
  Maintain Hope and Support while Confronting Reality

With the exception of needle phobia, all broadly applicable regardless of the child's age.

Get Your Head in Gear

When you fly on a commercial jetliner, you're told that in the event of an emergency, the oxygen masks will drop down and you should put yours on before assisting a child. That's the absolute rule in cancer caregiving when children are concerned, particularly in light of the loss of control that a cancer diagnosis provokes.

For many parents, the process of getting their own heads in gear begins with understanding what's happening and why. The randomness of the "why" is nearly impossible to accept, especially since parents are so inclined to wonder whether they could have done something to avoid it.

Jeff's mother recalled her reaction when her 13-year-old son was treated over 25 years ago for stage IVA Hodgkin's lymphoma:

> It was devastating. I was in denial and angry. What do you say when your kid asks, "Mommy, am I going to die?" How do you say you don't know? I remember him lying in the bed and just screaming because he was in such pain. You can't make it go away, you can't make it better. You're supposed to kiss the booboo and make it all go away. You'd trade places with him a million times over if you could, because you don't want to see your kid go through that kind of pain.

So expect the shock, figure out what you <u>can</u> control in day-to-day living, and be prepared to put away your frustration that control was yanked away from you. Your job is to assume as much control as you can by pinning down the diagnosis fast and advocating on the child's behalf during treatment.

The Nemours Foundation has published an article entitled "Childhood Cancer"[11] that may help provide parents with a foundation for understanding this phenomenon.

Pin Down and Understand the Diagnosis Fast

Some caregivers accuse the diagnostic process of moving too slowly. That can be especially true of a childhood illness. When a child shows initial symptoms, cancer often isn't the first thing that comes to a pediatrician's mind, especially when the symptoms present as something that could be caused by an infection, allergy, or persistent cold.

It often takes parental urgency, persistence, and even going to several different types of specialists to get the right answer:

- ❧ **Michael S's** rare medullary thyroid carcinoma manifested at first as sore throats, swollen glands, and fatigue.

- ❧ **Jeff's** Stage IV-A Hodgkin's Lymphoma at age 13 presented initially as persistent breathing problems, night sweats, and vomiting, appearing in random combinations as he lost considerable weight.

The parents of both children had a high sense of urgency and consulted with multiple specialists before getting their diagnoses pinned down. In contrast, four-year-old **Eric** had a lump near his collar bone that was visible, palpable, and easily identified as something out of the ordinary; his diagnosis of a rare and aggressive T-Cell Lymphoblastic Lymphoma took only 36 hours.

So your job as a caregiver of a potentially sick child is to demonstrate urgency and ensure that your medical team gets to the core of the problem quickly. Don't hesitate to cajole, nudge, insist, and even push with considerable force to get a clear and complete diagnosis and a viable treatment plan as swiftly as possible.

---

11 *www.kidshealth.org/parent/medical/cancer/cancer.html*

Again, the Nemours Foundation's guide explains how childhood cancer differs from the cancers that attack adults. It may prove useful to you as you become immersed in the diagnostic process.

Seek the Best Treatments

Children with cancer require different treatments than adults because their bodies are still developing and so many treatments (chemotherapy and radiation) can be toxic to different degrees. As a result, it is essential to seek out experts in your child's particular kind of cancer.

One of the most useful resources for doing so is the website for the Children's Oncology Group (COG),[12] which is the National Cancer Institute's clinical trials arm for children and adolescents. The locations index offers two invaluable tools:

- An address finder[13] for over 200 participating institutions to help you locate the pediatric cancer center at the children's hospital, university medical center, or cancer center closest to your home.
- A downloadable family handbook[14] that is available in English, Spanish, and French.

This website might well be the best first step after a cancer diagnosis for a family trying to figure out "What do we do now?" The Patients and Family tab offers links to medical information, insights about coping with childhood cancer, and information about research underway at over 200 sites. COG has a large consortium of research institutions that are funding and developing new therapies and fielding clinical trials for new treatments. While there are never enough such trials, children and adolescents have a far higher likelihood of being admitted to a clinical trial because there are fewer candidates for each trial.

---

12 *www.childrensoncologygroup.org/*
13 *www.childrensoncologygroup.org/index.php/locations/*
14 *www.childrensoncologygroup.org/index.php/cog-family-handbook*

The <u>American Cancer Society</u> also provides a sound general overview[15] of the kinds of issues that caregivers need to consider when a child or adolescent is diagnosed with cancer. Further, it offers a good rundown on <u>how to navigate the health system</u>[16] on your child's behalf. Finally, it has an index of the websites for leading pediatric cancer centers nationwide for gathering additional information about treatment options[17].

Conserve Your Energy

Predictable sleep and your normal routine will go away for a significant period of time. Eric, who was four, hadn't had many shots before his sudden diagnosis with a rare and aggressive T-Cell Lymphoblastic Lymphoma.

Despite his rapid lymphoma diagnosis and quick surgical intervention, **Eric's mother** was so physically and emotionally depleted that she had to be taken from the surgical waiting area to his hospital room in a wheelchair, where she and her husband cried in private. Post surgery, neither she nor her husband slept because the IV fluids had Eric up often, chemo medications had him vomiting, monitor wires tangled with his body when he turned in his sleep, and he cried every time people came into the room to check or inject him. It took several weeks before they settled into a routine that allowed both parents to get even half a night's uninterrupted sleep.

This is only a snippet of one family's experience at the outset of treatment, but it's illustrative of the strains—both physical and emotional—that accompany most childhood cancer diagnoses. So the lesson from these and other stories is make sure someone else is covering for you so you can take a deliberate breather to:

- ❧ Figure out a way to take turns so someone gets some sleep and has the emotional reserves to handle the day-to-day interactions

---

15   *www.cancer.org/treatment/childrenandcancer/whenyourchildhascancer/index*
16   *www.cancer.org/treatment/childrenandcancer/whenyourchildhascancer/ childrendiagnosedwithcancerunderstandingthehealthcaresystem/index*
17   *www.cancer.org/treatment/childrenandcancer/whenyourchildhascancer/ children-diagnosed-with-cancer-late-effects-of-cancer-treatment*

with the medical team, even if you have to trade off shifts 12 hours at a time.

- ∽ Take an hour or so every few days for yourself—a massage, a soak in a hot tub, some yoga. It may be easier said than done, but your emotional reservoir will empty quickly, and an hour here or there can restore your energy and patience if you can get someone you trust to cover for you during that short period.

- ∽ Take a short walk—to the cafeteria or gift shop, around the block, down the hall—or find an outdoor garden where you might just sit in the sun for 10 minutes with your eyes closed.

- ∽ Stop blaming yourself.

However short the respite, it will increase your resilience and effectiveness.

Advocate during Treatment

Most of the caregivers for cancer patients of any age explained the need to take a strong advocacy position in dealing with the medical system. It doesn't matter how good a hospital is. There are always things that fall through the cracks or get missed, especially when the staff shifts change.

As you begin coming to grips with the facts of the diagnosis, remember that you're the customer of the medical system and should be treated that way. When your instincts tell you that "business as usual" is taking too long without improving the symptoms, or that something is being missed, you should advocate for your patient and ask for, or even demand, a referral or a change in the process.

This is often hard for a parent to do well because caregiving for a child with cancer is such an emotional roller coaster. **Doug's mother** initially felt powerless when her 14-year-old son was being treated for Ewing's sarcoma:

> *When the medical team members were hurting him, I didn't know what to do. It made me feel helpless, but I didn't want to do more harm through my reaction. If his oncologist hadn't come in right then, I don't know what I'd have done. Observing it, we*

concluded we'd never EVER leave him by himself again. There were times when things were more predictable and you knew the staff on duty, but every time there could be an OMIGOD moment, we made sure we were present. It was a great comfort to him to know that someone was there.

Despite her own emotional distress, she recognized that she had to inject some control into the situation. She and her husband never left Doug alone thereafter when he was hospitalized, trading off as necessary to also care for Doug's brother at home. She also pushed back with the medical team when her instincts told her that something wasn't right.

Caregivers say that you must:

- ✎ Keep asking questions to ensure you know what is being done and why, and that it is being done with the least disruption to the patient.

- ✎ When your gut feeling is that something is wrong, push to speak to supervisors to ensure that professional caregiving is done as well as possible.

- ✎ Be willing to change hospitals or medical teams if you feel that you're not being treated as a valued partner or that something important is being missed.

Advocating hard doesn't mean losing your temper or giving medical professionals a difficult time. Your emotions are a natural companion to the situation in which you've been dropped, and the medical team will understand that. After all, who wouldn't be emotional in caring for a child battling cancer?

The problem is that some parents let their emotions hijack their minds when they're interacting with the medical team. They may become angry and agitated, which in turn may lead them to take out their frustration on the physicians and other team members inappropriately.

When Lanie, age nine, was having sustained headaches and started vomiting for no explainable reason, her mother pressed doctors for a clear diagnosis.

But getting that clarity took several months and trips to different medical providers. Finally, a specialized children's hospital determined that Lanie had a rare pilocytic astrocytoma tumor of the cerebellum, one so rare that there was only one other child in the world with the same tumor at the time. Perhaps as a result of the diagnostic delay and its associated stresses, **Lanie's mother** became an extreme advocate, losing her temper at the medical staff so often that she was nearly banned from her daughter's hospital.

A more constructive role model was **Samantha's mother**, who exhibited a calm style and collaborative approach with two-year-old Sam's medical team during her multi-year leukemia treatment:

> *I was determined to learn everything I could so I'd understand what was going on, could interpret the decisions her doctors were making, and could be part of the process. In the hospital, I was determined that I needed to know that the time there was being well used and that Samantha was being protected from infections by being kept there as short a time as possible. When I saw inefficiencies, I requested a meeting with the head nurse and whomever else she wanted to bring. I thought they'd say I was the mother from hell, but I didn't care.*
>
> *Instead of being angry or challenging me, they took everything down that I said and thanked me for taking the initiative. They made sure we had nurses that we had worked with before and would focus on us and be as efficient as they could.*

On one occasion, she conveyed to the nursing staff a suggestion from the nurse in the emergency room. By brokering a conversation between them, they were together able to cut a half-day of Samantha's in-hospital treatment time.

Once again, the bottom line on advocating is that if your gut tells you something isn't right, ask the professional caregivers to explain what they are doing and why, and to change it if necessary. If their answer isn't satisfactory, ask to see the supervising nurse or doctor. It's perfectly acceptable to do so and to work your way up the chain of command. Just be aware that your understandable concerns may prove counterproductive if you let them make you too intense and emotional to collaborate with the medical team.

Head Off Needle Phobia in Very Young Children

It's important to help children between the ages of 3 and 7 or so to adjust to getting needles several times a day. Eric, who was four, hadn't had many shots before his sudden diagnosis with a rare and aggressive T-Cell Lymphoblastic Lymphoma. He nearly became needle-phobic, even though he was being treated at one of the world's foremost children's hospitals. Sometimes the anxiety was stronger than the actual physical discomfort, but Eric's parents felt overwhelmed in their desire to reduce Eric's upset.

There are several strategies that might help in this kind of situation. One is providing rewards for every needle stick that is completed. This might be in the form of stickers or a citation of bravery in helping the medical team to treat the cancer. Two resources toward that end are:

    ❧ A bravery cape or stickers[18] (for purchase)

    ❧ Bravery certificates[19] (free)

In addition, if you're facing this very common challenge, ask your medical team about using a product to numb the skin and reduce sensations before giving shots. Leading products include Buzzy Cream[20] (a numbing cream with lidocaine anesthetic in it), EMLA[21] (a cream with lidocaine and prilocaine anesthetics), or Pain Ease[22] (a cream or spray that chills the skin to reduce sensations). Another interesting new product is the Buzzy Bee,[23] which uses cold and vibration to short-circuit pain sensations. Each hospital or medical team may have its preferences, or maybe you can actually teach *them* something.

---

18   *www.therapeuticpillows.com/brave-kid-capes/cape-kits/*
19   *www.123certificates.com/bravery.php*
20   *www.buzzy4shots.com/topical-anesthetics/*
21   *www.childrensmn.org/Manuals/PFS/Med/018866.pdf*
22   *www.gebauer.com/Products/Gebauer-s-Pain-Ease/gebauer---painease/*
23   *http://buzzy4shots.com/*

Fight Isolation

Feelings of isolation emerge almost immediately after a cancer diagnosis. People who haven't experienced the cancer journey can't imagine the degree to which both patient and caregiver may feel that no one else can understand the stresses and dislocations they're experiencing. Overcoming the inevitable, burdensome sense of loneliness can ease anxiety and offer a reality check for both caregivers and the child himself.

Shortly after her four-year-old son was diagnosed with a brain tumor, **Michael L's mother** met someone who helped ease her sense of isolation:

> *The night the pathology report was coming back, another little boy and his mother were in the room. She asked whether things were OK. My father said, "I'm really sorry, but we just found out that my grandson has a brain tumor, so we can't talk." She said, "Oh, my son has a brain tumor too."*
>
> *After I came back with the pathology report, my father introduced me to her. I fell into her lap, and she allowed me to cry for an hour. She's become my best friend. Fate brought us together that night. Knowing they were farther along in the process really helped. Somebody else had gone through the same nightmare.*

This connection with someone who understood didn't make the nightmare go away, but it gave Michael's mom a strong shoulder to lean on when things got rough during treatment. Both children are thriving today, and their mothers continue to be friends.

Children with cancer often experience unique issues with their social relationships. It's particularly hard for a parent to see his child's friends disappear because the friends don't understand their own fear and discomfort with the emotions surrounding cancer. **Michael S's father** saw that happen with his son:

> *Michael had been a good-looking kid and a star in the actors' guild at school, but after his surgery he looked like a refugee from a Frankenstein movie. He had three friends who stuck by him and became*

life-long friends. They stuck by him even when he was in the hospital, and they made sure he got to the senior prom.

A huge other group who were supposedly his friends fell away. We noticed it, too, with our friends. People who aren't used to personal crises back away and don't know how to deal with you.

Understanding "pull-aways" is harder for a child—especially a child with cancer. The message is that those who pull away probably weren't the friends you thought they were.

Parent caregivers can help their charges when that happens. **Doug's mother** realized early on in his treatment that her son was having trouble staying in touch with the aspects of his high school experience that had once defined his normal life:

Doug recovered from surgery without complications and resumed rigorous chemo. The medical team thought it better if he not return to school for his sophomore year, so we had him tutored at home. He missed his sports and friends, and he felt cut off. We saw signs that Doug was getting depressed. He craved normalcy, but it was out of reach. His life had been totally upended. So I helped him to re-establish his connections.

His mom's outreach was so successful that during Doug's last days three years later, his friends attended his brother's eighth-grade graduation in Doug's place, and they were at Doug's bedside when he died.

Plan for Survivorship Issues

According to Dana Farber Cancer Institute and Boston Children's Hospital, children's cancers are rare,[24] and survival rates are high. For children and adolescents diagnosed with cancer in the United States, they have risen dramatically, to an average of 85 percent in general and to over 90 percent for some childhood cancers.[25]

---

24   *www.danafarberbostonchildrens.org/For-Families/Childhood_Cancer_Facts.aspx*
25   *Ibid.*

Two issues generally confront caregivers as treatment draws to a close and survivorship evolves:

1. Most families, after the shock of the diagnosis and flurry of initial treatment activities, settle into a routine. They establish relationships with doctors, nurses and other caregivers, and become more comfortable that the child's situation is under control. Then, when active treatment stops, they often feel like their safety cocoon has been breached. Treatment routines and the daily contacts with the health care professionals no longer stabilize their lives. Further, parents may feel anxiety about how to recognize warning signs of a possible relapse and face a sense of isolation when friends and family who surrounded them during their health care crisis gradually return to their normal lives.

   The American Cancer Society's page on "When Your Child's Treatment Ends"[26] provides useful insights about what to expect and how to handle your after-treatment concerns.

2. Because pediatric cancers arise at times when the child's body is developing and most susceptible to damage from toxic therapies, it's important for caregivers to stay vigilant for what's called "late effects" of cancer treatment. Hopefully, the child will remain cancer-free for the rest of his or her life. But cancer therapies target fast-growing cells and may also damage healthy body parts that are still developing, like children's hearts, brains, and reproductive systems. The potential problems will show up later in life. I raise these issues not to scare you, but to help you enter the aftermath of cancer treatments with your eyes open. The American Cancer Society's information on that topic (downloadable from its website) can give you an overview of issues to watch for later in life and questions to ask of your child's medical team.[27]

---

26 www.cancer.org/treatment/childrenandcancer/whenyourchildhascancer/when-your-childs-treatment-ends
27 www.cancer.org/treatment/childrenandcancer/whenyourchildhascancer/children-diagnosed-with-cancer-late-effects-of-cancer-treatment

When the Child's Diagnosis is Grim:
Maintain Hope and Support While Confronting Reality

Children aren't supposed to die, but the harsh truth of cancer is that doesn't obey any rules about what's rational or fair. When a child is seriously ill and at risk of dying, you need particularly effective and sensitive guidance. An excellent resource is the booklet "*What Do We Do Now?*" by Quality of Life Publishing (QoL). It provides an overview of how to handle the key issues, as well as offering a list of other reference resources on the topic. In general the content parallels the ideas and examples offered in this book, but with a special focus on the age of the patient. Most of QoL's publications are made available to institutions in the form of "branded" booklets, but you can access a single copy by calling 877-513-0099 or going to the company's website, *www.QoLpublishing.com.*

Doug's mother offers some helpful tactics for engaging a dying child in productive dialogue based on the insights and experience she had during her son's last days:

> One thing I learned not to ask was, "How are you feeling?," but instead to ask, "What are you thinking about?" It provoked some wonderful conversations. Keep a journal. I kept a separate journal documenting conversations along the way as he was dying, separate from the medical journal.
>
> Doug was on morphine and was lucid till the last day or two. He could interact with his buddies. In fact, they were there so often that parents would apologize if their kid couldn't come. The school waived final exams for four of them. Doug died on the last day of school.
>
> On his final day, before he died, I asked Doug how he wanted to be remembered. I also read comments to him from the notes people had written to him in his yearbook. It was one of the hardest things I had to do, but it was a gift to him.

Help Siblings Cope with Survivor Guilt

Cancer isn't a rational disease. There's often no clear reason why one patient makes it through and another dies. Rather than trying to explain it to a child experiencing survivor guilt, all you can do is express your relief that your child was one of the lucky ones. The issues are even more complex if another child has died.

Jeff overcame his childhood Hodgkin's lymphoma. Yet one of the most impactful experiences for **Jeff's mother**, in the aftermath of his "re-birthday" bone marrow transplant, was seeing how Jeff reacted to learning that other children whom he had befriended during his treatment didn't survive their cancers:

> *I remember Jeff sitting on the kitchen floor sobbing as he asked, "Mom, why not me?" One of the hardest things for me was when Jeff was leaving the hospital, after his transplant. One of his friends, a boy his same age, had leukemia and was terminal. It tore me up to say good-bye to this friend and his mother when I knew I was taking my son home and he was going to be fine, but this boy wouldn't.*

These kinds of feelings can be even more severe when it's a sibling who is sick. For a caregiver, no act can be more important than:

- ❦ Acknowledging their distress and strained emotions to demonstrate that you understand how they feel.

- ❦ Helping them understand that cancer is a random disease and that there's no explaining why one patient survives and another doesn't.

- ❦ Emphasizing that you love them and are eager to offer whatever support you can in working through those feelings.

- ❦ Helping them to think about things they might do to help support others who are feeling vulnerable as a result of this happening.

Help Healthy Siblings Avoid Feelings of Neglect

When one child in a family has cancer, the other siblings may need special attention. Caregivers say that it's too easy to focus all of your waking energy on the sick child. Depending on their age, engaging healthy siblings in caring for the one who has cancer can help to both manage their expectations and let them know how much you love and trust them. Even though their daily life has been severely disrupted, try to sustain routines that will help the healthy siblings to preserve whatever remnants of normalcy they can.

Jeff's mother still remembers that early on in his treatment for Hodgkin's lymphoma, she got an earful from his sister:

> One day my daughter, who was 16, asked, "Mom, do I have to get sick too to get your attention? Because I'm not here anymore." You're so focused on the child who is sick, I don't know how families who have multiple children do it. You say to yourself, "Whoa! Thank God she was in tune enough with her feelings to say it." She did both of us a favor. She helped me realize that I needed to pay more attention to her needs too. After that, we set aside one night a week to do something together, even though Jeff was hospitalized or recovering at home. We'd go to a movie, shopping, or out with her friends. We left her father in charge of her brother.

Some families learned the hard way how important it was to establish a support network for their healthy children. When Michael S was diagnosed with a rare cancer during his senior year of high school, his sister—then a high school junior—was determined not to add to the burden facing her parents. **Michael S's** father explains that:

> His sister had been to almost every doctor's appointment with Michael and was fully in the loop that his cancer could be very serious. She tried to be strong for everyone and put up an "I'm fine" wall as her own defense mechanism. We knew this could happen, but we had so much on our hands that it was easy to take her at face value. Then one day, she had a complete meltdown in school. That was our first visible sign of how much she had been hurting.

Then we learned that we needed others in the family tested because Michael's cancer was hereditary. As a result, my wife was diagnosed six months later with a related cancer. Right away, having learned from our first episode and knowing that Michael was still in treatment, we set up a support system for our daughter without telling her. We talked with a teacher, guidance counselor, and the directors of both the chorus and the band, people with whom she would have frequent access. During my wife's treatment, our daughter visited the guidance counselor frequently (sometimes daily) to discuss concerns she didn't want to raise with us. Afterward, she acknowledged that these support resources had been enormously helpful in sustaining her equilibrium.

These stories illustrate that both carving out time to spend with the other children in the family and ensuring that they have their own support network are critical elements in helping the healthy siblings make it through the cancer experience with minimal damage.

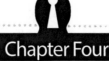

Chapter Four

When Children Lose a Parent or Sibling to Cancer

Coaching children through the death of a parent or sibling is something that few people get to practice before it happens. For most of us, it's an event that happens during adulthood, so it's hard to explain to a child because it's such a shock and lasts forever. The experience may differ based on whether the death was anticipated and there was time to help prepare the children, or it was sudden. In the end, the challenge for remaining caregivers is to help children understand and deal with the loss at the same time they are dealing with their own grief.

This chapter addresses how to:

- ✑ **Help Prepare Children for a Death**
- ✑ **Let Children Help Ease the Dying Process**
- ✑ **Recognize Children's Reactions and Real Concerns**
- ✑ **Help Children Understand Your Need to Build a New Normal**

Help Prepare Children for a Death

The most valuable resources in preparing caregivers for the dying process can be hospice professionals and the publications they offer. In addition, there are several resources where end-of-life issues are addressed, including:

- ॐ *The Little Blue Book* is available in several forms. One is called *Gone From My Sight*.[28] This version is written by Barbara Karnes, an experienced hospice nurse and trainer.

- ॐ *Final Gifts*[29] by Maggie Callanan and Patricia Kelley, Bantam Books, 1993 (Paperback, 239 pages) was cited by several caregivers as having been invaluable in understanding the importance of nonverbal communication with someone who is dying.

- ॐ The American Cancer Society[30] offers helpful short and downloadable information about grief and loss.

There's nothing more difficult than saying good-bye to someone you care about who is dying. A number of the caregivers, however, talk about the importance of not having regrets, especially for children. They urge making sure you and they have the opportunity say everything you want to say to the person before he dies and that you and the children have those important memories. Because hearing is the last sense to go, you can share an important message even very near the end. You can't say it too soon, but if you wait, it might just become too late.

For **Jacqueline's husband**, it was important that all of the children got the opportunity to say good-bye to their mom:

They kept her alive so my sons could come in from Japan to say good-bye. I really appreciated that. Jacqueline wasn't conscious but she wasn't dead. We all talked to her. Everyone got the chance to say good-bye. It was consoling for all of us. I provided all of her care, with no hospice. What was hard was to look at someone you

---

28 www.GoneFromMySight.com
29 www.maggiecallanan.com/finalgifts.htm
30 www.cancer.org/treatment/treatmentsandsideeffects/emotionalsideeffects/griefandloss/index

love and realize she's dying. You want to show her how much you love her and to make that transition as comforting and as painless as possible.

Journals, letters, or even recorded personal messages from the patient to loved ones can offer a permanent record for them to read at key milestones later on. Saying good-bye in written or recorded form is a thoughtful gift that some dying patients provide for the consolation of their loved ones after they are gone. It gives the survivors something they can review and cherish in their low moments. For more guidance on how to say good-bye, *www.caring.com* is a good resource.

Both experts and caregivers say that confronting feelings of helplessness in the face of a pending death is an important part of acceptance and realizing that you can't change the outcome. Doing so can help ease the impact on children.

Unfortunately hindsight is perfect on this topic. **Deborah O's husband** and family had difficulty confronting the likelihood of her death 9 months after her diagnosis with Stage 4 inoperable lung cancer. He actually searched the house several times in the wake of her death in the hopes of finding good-bye messages from her. In hindsight, he has come to realize that for her, saying good-bye may have felt like being unfaithful to the family's hopes and prayers. He suggests that patients:

> *be encouraged to say good-bye before they become too ill to do so, even if it turns out to be like the Rolling Stones Farewell Tour which, I think, has been underway since the early 1990s.*

In the late stages of her husband's life, **Tim's wife** tried to ensure that his death would not be more devastating than necessary for their children:

> *There's a point where it's almost not about the person who dies. It's more about what will make it OK for the ones who live. It doesn't mean you have to tell the kids he's going to die, but you have to say, "He's really sick and having lots of problems right now, and his heart is really weak." At that point they might ask, "Is he going to die?" and I'd say, "I hope not, but it's possible. He could die." That was really important for the kids to hear.*

Joe's wife described how she and Joe tried to help the children confront the fact that he was dying:

> A few weeks before he died, Joe had been in the hospital with pneumonia and on bypass. Our younger son Matthew absolutely refused to come to the hospital or to talk about it. He was a senior in high school. He was the heartbreak kid right there. Joe was his best friend in the world.
>
> Shortly before he died, Joe said, "I don't think I can keep doing this, but I don't want my boys to think I'm a quitter." I told Matthew he had to go see his dad because I thought Daddy was going to die. There he was, a six-foot, 17-year-old kid, and he just collapsed in his daddy's arms. Joe talked to Matthew about sports, which they both loved. He said, "I expect that when you have kids, you'll go out there and coach them, just like I coached you. Do what you want to do, and be what you want to be." Joe died about 36 hours later. I firmly believe that Joe waited until they had had that conversation to die.

Many experts say that people who are dying work to ensure that they will complete "unfinished business" before they let go to the dying process. That was certainly the case for Joe.

Let Children Ease the Patient's Dying Process

Sometimes children can actually play an invaluable role in a patient's dying process. They take their lead from their parents about handling and preparing for a loved one's death. To the degree that you can encourage them to interact with the patient during his decline, they will be left with far less unfinished business. They are likely to ask questions even if they aren't told explicitly what is happening, so it may be useful to decide when and how to share information, rather than waiting to react to questions that might arise at awkward times.

Artie's daughter-in-law coached her children ages eight and five through their grandfather's dying process, as Artie was being cared for in their home:

We set up hospice way before we needed it. The woman from hospice would come and do arts and crafts with the kids, what she called "heart play." They talked about how Papa was dying, and she suggested a wonderful thing for them to do. She asked, "Do you want to make a memory box and windmill, so every time you see it blow, you can think that's Papa with you?" She was laying the groundwork for the healing process afterward.

I had been so nervous about the kids, but we had them come in while he was dying to give Artie hugs and kisses. They said their good-byes. It was tremendously stressful, but having him die at home was the most rewarding thing we could have done.

The night after he died, I thought I was going to have a problem getting our son back into his room, so we offered to move his own bed back in there right away, but they both climbed into the hospital bed and went to sleep. They still have a pillowcase that they call "Papa's pillowcase," and they have it in a baggie so it still smells like Papa. They still fight over who gets to sleep with Papa. They came up with that themselves.

The woman from hospice came back three or four times after Artie died. They filled the memory box right after and put the windmill on the mailbox. The memory box says "I love Papa" on it. It's filled with little things: One of his mints, his watch, his wallet—just little things.

For this family, and for many others, being open with the kids allowed them to to enrich the patient's dying moments and to sustain positive memories that helped everyone in the household.

Recognize Children's Reactions and Real Concerns

Children usually react to the loss of a parent or sibling with sadness, uncertainty, and fear. The sadness is for loss of what they knew, the uncertainty is about what life will be like without that parent or sibling, and the fear is that remaining family members might also die. Learning to get beyond the constant sense of emptiness may seem like an overwhelming task.

Tim's wife explained that her children have had a difficult time in the period since Tim died:

> *When he died, I was numb. Then I started to cry all the time, loudly. The kids understood that I grieved. They grieved too. My younger one had her therapist to help. My older daughter didn't start to grieve until this past summer, after she got out of high school. She wanted to be like every other normal kid and didn't tell anyone. She didn't want to be different, to be the kid whose father had died. Both of them put how they really felt about it on hold for a while.*
>
> *The kids were 12 and 15 when he died, and they're 16 and 19 now. It hasn't been easy. You just put one foot ahead of the other and try to make the right decisions every day with your kids and yourself. It still isn't easy. My entire life is completely different and will never ever be the same.*

Part of the difficulties lie in the fact that grief can take so many different, unexpected forms. After **Doug**, died, his younger brother Brandon by two years found it hard to adjust, as his mother describes:

> *Brandon wanted normalcy for himself, but he went to the high school where Doug had been king. Teachers and everyone there knew Doug. He was in Doug's realm but wanted to hide so he could be Brandon. He changed his friends; those who had been his best buddies were left behind. They were still nice kids that he chose, but he got more into marijuana, etc. We discovered it from his behaviors.*
>
> *Conversation was really important at that time. Brandon was worried about us. He could hear us crying at night and didn't want to worry us, so he tried to power through. The magic of conversation was knowing what times of day would work best for him. He tended not to talk at meals, but late at night or in the car were the more receptive times for him. It turns out that Brandon worried that he'd get cancer when he got to be 14.*

Brandon later went to a local state university. He lives at home and has developed a nice relationship with his parents, who are getting used to him as an adult. Doug's brother is healthy and getting happier.

While everyone grieves differently, interviewees suggested some things to do that can help ease both caregivers' and children's pain and sense of loss:

- ⊱ Participating in a grief counseling group (sometimes called bereavement groups) can allow connecting to other caregivers who have shared a similar experience and may make them feel less alone.

- ⊱ Writing down stories of good times that might have been shared in the patient's final days gives something tangible and positive to recall when you're feeling most alone.

- ⊱ For older children and adults, keeping a journal of your feelings and experiences may help you get a grip on them. For younger children, the parallel might be drawing, coloring, or painting pictures that remind them of the person they've lost or good times they had together.

In many cases, when a child's feelings about the death of a parent aren't dealt with candidly, they may not surface until many years later.

Margaret and Bill's son lost both of his parents to cancer, his mother when he was in high school and his father four years later. In fact, he didn't even learn that she had been treated for cervical cancer until he read it on her death certificate years later. He never had the opportunity to confront his own grief until he helped a friend whose father was dying:

> *I relived the death of both of my parents through a friend whose father was diagnosed with leukemia. He was devastated. I was going to the hospital or staying with him at the house every few days for nearly nine months. I sat with his dad when he was on a respirator. I relived and felt for the first time what it was like to be a caregiver.*
>
> *My friend expressing his raw emotions was the total opposite of the way I had motored on. I needed that. It helped me let my*

45

emotions out. Now I'm not ashamed of crying. I suppressed so much when my mother died.

Losing a parent is a unique and difficult experience after you've been to college and left home, in part because there aren't a lot of support resources for that age group. That was the situation for **Claire's daughter** after her mother died of lung cancer:

> *When you're a teenage girl, you're always bickering with your mother. Then you're away at college for four years. At that point, my mother became my friend. For those couple of years when she was well, we did things together as adults. She had had a difficult life. She was happy and finally starting to enjoy life, and she no longer had a young child to worry about. I never got to spend enough time with her as my friend.*
>
> *It's probably the most difficult thing I'll ever go through in my life. Nothing else could be that bad. I still have days when I feel sorry for myself because she's not around, and I'll be sad that she'll never get to see what I've done.*

For teenagers and young adults who lose a parent before or in the midst of forming adult relationships with them, there remains a void. It's described as a hole that feels like the absence of a relationship they had hoped they would have and the lack of a nurturing adult presence in their lives.

Joe's wife, who is a nurse in the hospital where he died, found that handling Joe's death was especially hard for her younger son, who was still in high school when his father died:

> *Matthew hasn't moved on very well. I've told him that he and his daddy had more good times together in a few years than some people do in a lifetime, and he knows that. Matthew is still at a point of not wanting to get that close again to anyone and get hurt again. A piece of that boy's soul left that day.*

For older children, grief may take longer to heal. For **Nora and George's daughter**, the challenge was the duration of her grief—how long it took her to process the loss of her parents, even though her mother died more than 15 years before her father:

> *The biggest frustration was that I thought, "I'll get through this in two or three months. In two or three months I'll be able to navigate my emotions and feelings." I thought I'd be the same person I was before. That's very naïve. The reality is that healing takes many many many years. That's one of the key things to learn, that the mourning continues and you grow because of the experience. The mourning never ends.*

Help Children Understand Your Need to Build A New Normal

Figuring out what the new normal will look like after the death of a family member is always a challenge, but even more so when the widowed parent seeks out another life companion. Interestingly, older children seem to have a harder time accepting that "getting-on-with-life" decision than younger ones.

Didier's wife has been rebuilding her life for nearly five years, after losing her husband when she had a three-year-old and was about to give birth to their second child. Her children don't remember their father's death, so the healing and lifestyle redesign was hers to perform. She was adamant that she would not marry again. Now she's on the verge of marrying someone whom the children adore. She was a harder sell for him than the kids were!

Before Jacqueline died, she encouraged her husband to find another female companion. Even though he didn't deliberately set out to date after her death, serendipity struck, and he found a wonderful woman who fills part of the hole that Jacqueline left behind. What **Jacqueline's husband** didn't expect was how challenging the conversation with his adult children would be after he decided he wanted to marry again:

> *The kids gave me a rough time. My current wife helped me so much going through that process It took a good three years to win*

47

them over. They had a very difficult time seeing me with another woman. Before we got married two years ago, I went to Japan and personally asked my sons to come to the wedding. They did, but I know it had to hurt them.

We talked about that. "Here's the thing you have to remember," I said. "I loved your mother very much, and I went out of my way to do everything I could for her. The good Lord took her, and there's nothing I could do about that. She wanted me to be happy. I can't live alone. I need someone to talk to. Someone to have dinner with. Someone to cook for."

In contrast to Jacqueline's husband, who waited until the adult children bought in before remarrying, **Deborah O's husband** met someone special within several months after Deborah's death. He felt it represented no disloyalty because he had another child at home and had to get on with his life. When his older children gave him a hard time about marrying again so soon, he decided to move ahead anyway, telling them *"I loved your mother, but she's no longer here, and I have a right to have a life."* Now, nearly a year after the remarriage, the blended family is doing well, and his new wife has become another parent figure for his youngest son. She'll never replace his mother, but she's providing him with the family stability that he desperately needs.

Recovering after the death of a child is even more difficult than healing after a parent or spouse's death. Siblings may experience lasting pain and survivor guilt, and parents may be challenged to attend to the needs of surviving children as they deal with their own grief. Be prepared for sadness to erupt when you least expect it, but also remember to seek help in managing the healing process.

Experienced counseling resources for helping manage grief are often available through major pediatric cancer centers and cancer support organizations. These professionals can suggest ways of remembering the good times and creating or joining activities that will honor the deceased while nourishing those who are left behind. Additional resources are suggested in Chapter Five.

Other Resources for Caregivers Concerned about Children

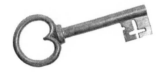

Most resources for caregivers on the topic of engaging the children recommend the approach that many of the interviewees shared—telling the truth but moderating how much you say based on their age, and recognizing that each child will handle that information differently. The sections below address:

- ⮞ **General Informational Resources**
- ⮞ **Support During and After Treatment**
- ⮞ **Support Specifically for Young Adults**
- ⮞ **Grief Support Resources—for Adults and for Children**

General Informational Resources

- ⮞ **American Childhood Cancer Association**[31] Cancer is the number one disease killer of children, and for those who survive, treatments are aggressive and may cause enormous

---

31   *www.acco.org/*

suffering. The ACCA provides information and support for children and adolescents with cancer and their families, to provide grassroots leadership through advocacy and awareness and to support research leading to a cure for all children diagnosed with this life-threatening disease.

∽ **Cancer Knowledge Network**[32] The Cancer Knowledge Network publishes a website that provides information and support, drawing on medical, support, and caregiver perspectives. Its newsletters and resource pool are impressive. Based in Canada, this is an organization operated by parents who have experienced childhood cancers.

∽ The **American Cancer Society**[33] provides ideas about how to involve and inform children about a cancer diagnosis in the family. Useful links and downloadable information are also available about how to tell a child that he or she has cancer.

Support During and After Treatment

There are several resources that provide respite activities to boost children's confidence and give the family unit relief from the day-to-day stresses of treatment. They represent a different form of support resource that many families find to be invaluable:

∽ **Camp Kesem**[34] is a nationwide network of 41 camps founded with the support of the LiveStrong Foundation.[35] These camps are created by students from universities who fund and run the camp program for children ages 6 to 18 who have a parent battling cancer, in remission, or who has died of cancer. The students raise all of the funds necessary to provide the camp experience at no cost to the campers. The students are unpaid but do this to provide respite and support to children who have had to grow up too soon as a result of parental cancer.

32 cancerkn.com/category/caregivers/
33 www.cancer.org/cancer/cancerinchildren/index
34 www.campkesem.org/
35 www.livestrong.org

For the summary of a Boston Globe article about a Camp Kesem in New Hampshire that is run by MIT students and alumni, see Camp Kesem Bella English Article (August 27, 2013).[36]

❧ **Camp Sunshine**[37] is located in Casco, Maine, on the shores of Sebago Lake. This program provides respite, support, joy and hope to children with life-threatening illnesses and their immediate families through all stages of their illness. It is a free year-round program that includes 24-hour onsite medical and psychosocial support. Bereavement programs are also offered. Many other such camps exist nationwide.

❧ **Magical Moon Foundation**[38] (MMF) is an organization that focuses on creating positive and empowering experiences for children and their families fighting cancer. Children who visit here are knighted into a fellowship of brave young knights who collaborate in a mission to build a "healthy Earth Kingdom where children won't get cancer." Through their shared activities at the farm and their individual projects, the knights provide mutual support and encouragement as they work through the difficult experience of cancer treatment.

MMF serves children nationwide, empowering them to find the warrior within. Rather than kids fighting cancer, they become brave young Knights turning their struggles into motivation. Each Knight pursues a project to help build a healthy Earth Kingdom where children won't get cancer. Michael L, who is now a teen-ager, found the experience uplifting and highly supportive.

Even if you don't find a camp like this in your area, these sites can provide ideas about activities or organizations that may be able to help provide needed support for kids.

---

36   www.boston.com/lifestyle/2013/08/26/summer-camp-for-kids-who-have-parent-with-cancer/d5zrrr9c8bFZpOzCOGYKAN/story.html
37   www.campsunshine.org/
38   www.magicalmoon.org/

Support Specifically for Young Adults

The issues for young adults facing cancer and their caregivers are particularly challenging for two reasons. First, it's often slow for young adults to get a timely and accurate diagnosis because symptoms may be subtle or unusual to see in patients in this age range. Second, there are unpredictable rest-of-your-life issues like fertility and long-term effects of aggressive therapies that may face survivors and their loved ones. As a result, some resources are particularly relevant for this population.

๛ **Stupidcancer.org.**[39] This site is particularly helpful for teens and young adults. It provides a variety of resources and sources of information and support. In its own words:

Stupidcancer.org empowers young adults affected by cancer through innovative and award-winning programs and services. We are the nation's largest support community for this underserved population and serve as a bullhorn for the young adult cancer movement. Our charter is to ensure that no one goes unaware of the age-appropriate support resources they are entitled to so they can get busy living.

Young adults, a largely unknown group in the war on cancer, account for 72,000 new diagnoses each year. That's one every eight minutes. It's also seven times more than all pediatric cancers combined. This is not OK!

๛ **LiveSTRONG Young Adult Alliance.**[40] Cancer in adolescents and young adults (ages 15-29) is often underrecognized and therefore diagnosed at fairly advanced stages. It usually requires aggressive advocacy with the medical system and persistence in pressing for explanations for physical conditions (that may present as constant colds, "permanent flu," or unexplained pain or discomfort) that aren't responding to initial treatments. This site provides information and resources to

---

39   *www.stupidcancer.org*
40   *www.livestrong.org/what-we-do/our-actions/programs-partnerships/*
     livestrong-young-adult-alliance/

help in understanding the medical, psychological, and emotional challenges facing this age group.

❧ **Team Shan.**[41] Team Shan is a nonprofit organization based in Ontario, Canada, which was created in the wake of Shannon Larsen's death of inflammatory breast cancer at age 24. Her mother Lorna discovered that medical professionals didn't recognize Shan's symptoms soon enough to catch the disease while it was still treatable. In response, she created Team Shan with the mission of educating the public, health care professionals, and young women about early detection, risk reduction, and prevention of breast cancer. The website includes a helpful literature review and information about public education campaigns conducted across Canada.

❧ **First Descents.**[42] This organization serves anyone between the ages of 18-39 who has heard the words, "You have cancer." They offer free outdoor adventure programs (including whitewater kayaking, rock climbing, mountaineering, and surfing) in eleven states, Canada, and South America. Some young survivor "graduates" call it the best week of their lives.

❧ **Survive and Thrive Expeditions (Canada).**[43] This organization aims to help young survivors "reflect, refocus, rebuild, and live." To quote from its website, *"Many young adults feel they have missed out on some of the best years of their lives and feel intense pressure to 'get on with it' once they have finished treatments. They often jump right back on the path they were following pre-diagnosis, just to realize that so much has changed and what they thought was important to them is not so important anymore."*

The travel, adventure, and in-depth reflection and exploration of the cancer episode is designed to allow survivors to give themselves permission to reflect on the past while refocusing on their current lives and to move forward with deeper insights about themselves.

---

41   *www.teamshan.ca/*
42   *www.firstdescents.org/*
43   *www.survivethrive.org/*

Grief Support Resources—for Adults

There are a number of resources that can help both in dealing with grief and in figuring out how to redeploy the energy that was going into the cancer fight. For an adult caregiver, these resources may be critically important in dealing with their own grief so they can help the children to do so as well:

- ◆ The **National Cancer Institute**,[44] also part of the NIH, has a fairly comprehensive website and describes various stages of grief, beginning at the point where a patient's death is anticipated. Try "bereavement" in the search engine.

- ◆ The **U.S. Library of Medicine**,[45] part of the National Institutes of Health (NIH), supports a website dedicated to helping people understand and deal with their feelings of grief. Go to the site and enter "bereavement" in the search engine.

- ◆ **Elizabeth Kübler-Ross** is famous for her work on death and dying. A summary of her work and her available books can be found at *www.grief.com*.[46] On the same website, David Kessler addresses practical issues, like how to handle holidays after a loved one's death.

- ◆ For those whose grief is becoming debilitating, the **Mayo Clinic**[47] offers help. Type "complicated grief" into the search engine.

- ◆ An excellent resource cited in Chapter Three is the booklet, *"What Do We Do Now?,"* by **Quality of Life Publishing (QoL)**. Most of QoL's publications are made available to institutions in the form of "branded" booklets, but you can access a single copy by calling 877-513-0099 or by visiting the company's website, *www.QoLpublishing.com.*

- ◆ Finally, one last resource may be helpful for those who are seeking a longer case study about how one family dealt with

---

44 *www.cancer.gov/cancertopics*
45 *www.nlm.nih.gov*
46 *www.grief.com*
47 *www.mayoclinic.com*

preparing the children for a parent's death. **How We Said Goodnight**,[48] a memoir by Rachel Silsdorf, discusses how she and her husband Arlan involved their two children as the family was anticipating his impending death.

Grief Support Resources—for Children

The most effective resources for children are often delivered close to home and in a home-like setting. To find such support, there are several clearing house sites:

- ❧ **The Family Bereavement Resource Manual**[49] (downloadable free in pdf form and published by Full Circle Grief Counseling) offers an extensive educational resource for understanding how to help children of varying ages to deal with their grief when a loved one dies. The Resources tab on Full Circle's website offers lists of websites and books that can be helpful in dealing with grief in children.

- ❧ The National Association of School Psychologists has issued a four-page downloadable document entitled "**Helping Children Cope with Loss, Death, and Grief: Tips for Teachers and Parents**."[50]

- ❧ The **Children's Grief Education Association**[51] provides a collection of documents in downloadable pdf format that offer guidance on such issues as whether children should go to funerals and how to tell them that a loved one has died. There is also a downloadable bibliography of resources, classified into age groups.

- ❧ Three individuals from **Ohio University** (Brad A. Imhoff, Kaela Vance, and Amberle Quackenbush)[52] have documented a series

---

48 *www.amazon.com*
49 *www.fullcirclegc.org/resources/fc_manual_feb11.pdf*
50 *www.nasponline.org/resources/crisis_safety/griefwar.pdf*
51 *www/childgrief.org/childgrief.htm*
52 *www.allohiocc.org/Resources/Documents/AOCC%202012%20Session%2062.pdf*

of activities that can help children who are grieving. Explanations are clear, and the nature of the activities is easy to implement at home.

∽ The **Dougy Center** (The National Center for Grieving Children and Families) is a resource to help you find bereavement counseling across the country.[53]

These resources should give you a sense for the kinds of information and support that is available "out there."

What's important is using such resources to help you and your loved ones to regain your sense of **control**, gather information that can help build **hope**, break down your feelings of **isolation**, and restore some sense of **normalcy** in your cancer-affected lives. You'll be able to keep your CHIN up in facing your own caregiving roller coaster because you'll know that the kids will be OK.

---

53   *www.dougy.org/*